Diarrhea: How to Stop Diarrhea Chronic or Severe

"Special Diarrhea Remedies and Diet"

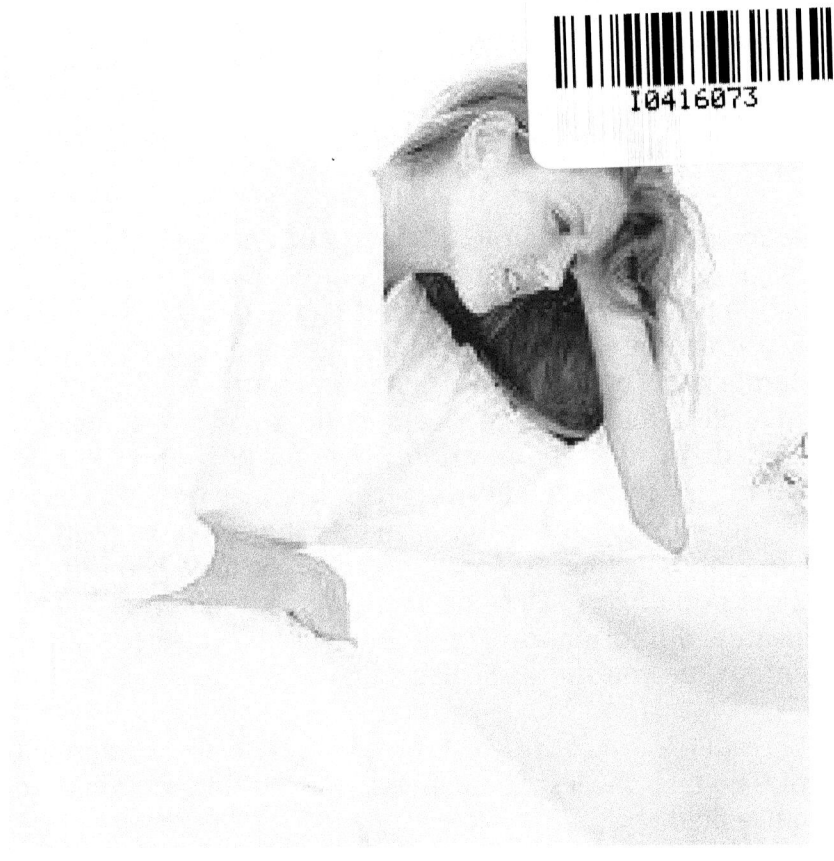

By Rudy S Silva, Natural Nutritionist

Table of Contents

1: Introduction - What Causes Diarrhea

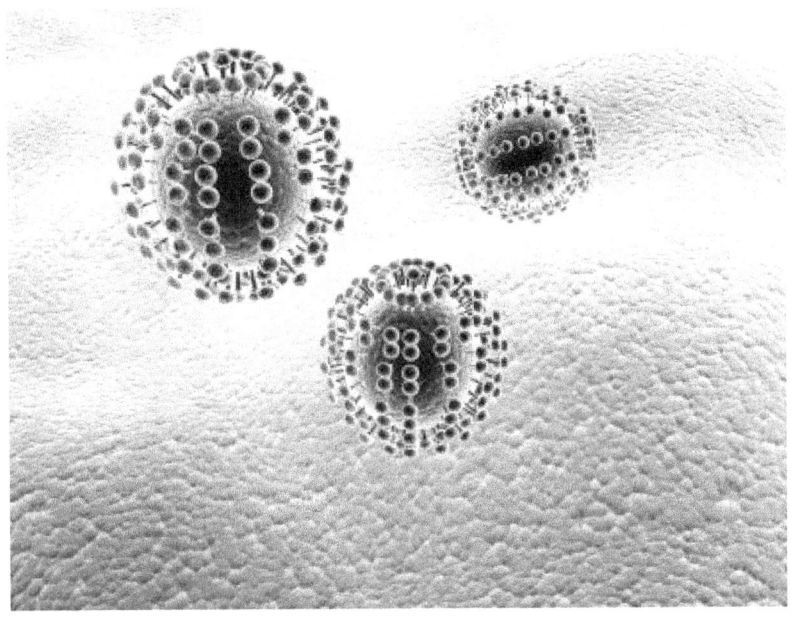

Get one of my best kindle books *free* by **clicking here.**

In this short book, you will find the foods, natural remedies and supplements that you need to stop or eliminate your diarrhea. There is not a lot of fluff here, so you will be able to get started right away on getting yourself back to normal.

Keep in mind that if you have chronic diarrhea, you should consult with your doctor.

When you have diarrhea, your body is secreting large amount of fluids in an effort to get rid of toxins, bacteria, and other foreign bodies.

Many times, diarrhea is not a life-threatening condition, and it can pass in a few days. When it persists for more than 2 to 4 days, you should see your doctor to make sure it is not a reflection of a more serious illness.

Now, first, you need to know some of the causes of diarrhea. If you can discover the cause of your diarrhea, hopefully you can avoid your diarrhea from getting worse or from returning.

What Causes Diarrhea

Some of the causes of typical diarrhea are nervous anxiety, poor eating habits, poor food combinations, pathogens, and certain types of food poisoning.

Diarrhea can also be caused by dysentery, which is a digestive infection caused by a parasite, such as an amoeba. In this condition, you can have bleeding that shows up in your stools. Bleeding can also occur with other types of diarrhea.

Diarrhea can also be caused, for some people, when they eat certain foods, such as restaurant fries, chocolate, and other foods. Many times your diarrhea can be cause by eating certain food at a restaurant. Restaurants typically use additives, such as sulfites as a preservative for the food they prepare in advance.

Here are more reasons you might have diarrhea:

- Allergic reaction to certain foods
- Celiac disease
- Inflammatory bowel disease
- Intestinal bacterial, candida, or viral infection
- Irritable bowel syndrome
- Lactose intolerance
- Parasites
- Reaction to artificial sweeteners
- Reaction to certain drugs
- Diabetes
- Viral or parasitic infections

- Cohn's disease
- Ulcerative colitis
-

Typically, you get diarrhea when food or meat is improperly handled, causing it to be contaminated with bacteria. This can happen in home or restaurant cooking.

Drugs

If you frequently use antibiotics, this will kill your internal good bacteria, and this can be a cause of diarrhea.

Disease of the colon

Colitis, an inflammation of the intestinal wall, irritable bowel syndrome, diverticulitis, and colon cancer can cause diarrhea.

Caffeine and Sensitivities

If you have a sensitive digestion system, simply drinking too much caffeine can give diarrhea. Caffeine is found in many products, such as tea, sodas, chocolate, and some drugstore products.

Stomach or colon irritation caused by excessive alcohol, sugar, salt, food additives, aspirin, NSAIDs, anti-inflammatory medication, or nicotine exposure can give you diarrhea.

Stomach acid

When you don't have enough stomach acid, you could develop diarrhea that shows up in the morning as loose stools or as recurring flatulence, after eating. If you use acid reducers to battle acid reflux, your stomach acid strength will be compromised.

Drug store products that decrease your stomach acid levels are dangerous products. if you use them frequently, they will cause you nutritional deficiency.

Allergies

Certain allergies and food sensitivities can cause diarrhea, such as milk and sugar. You need to avoid drinking fruit juices that contain sugar.

2: What to do for Diarrhea

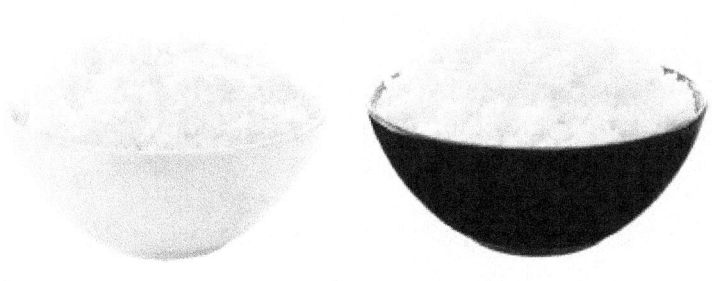

In most cases of acute diarrhea, you will get over it by yourself. By using the remedies and supplements listed in this book, you will get past diarrhea much faster. This is important, especially if you have a job or other activities that you need to attend to.

However, if you have acute, severe, or prolonged diarrhea, you will want to drink certain fluids to replace the electrolytes – ionic minerals – that you lose during your sickness. If you are unable to drink, these fluids, they will need to be replaced intravenously.

When you have diarrhea, don't take any type of commercial medication that stops diarrhea, since your body is eliminating whatever is irritating your intestinal tract. However, an antibacterial may be necessary, if this is the cause of your diarrhea.

It is ok to take gentle herbal remedies, teas, soups, and other natural remedies as outline in the book.

Here are a few things to get you started, when you have diarrhea. Many more food and remedy suggestions follow in the next chapters.

Drink Water, tea, or juices

Drink some fluids, so you don't get dehydrated, don't overdo it. Children become easily dehydrated with diarrhea. Drink teas, such as chamomile, raspberry, slippery elm, or ginger, which are described in later chapters.

It's ok to sip carob powder stirred in hot water. You can also make a green drink, by mixing one teaspoon of liquid chlorophyll, the juice of one lemon squeezed, and a cup of water. If you have a super green power, use this and add some honey to sweeten it up.
Keep hydrated with lots of low-sugar, no-sugar, and low-sodium fluids.

Rice Water

Drink diluted rice water. Here's how to make it. Boil 1 cup of rice with 4 cups of water for 45 minutes, strain and add a pinch of salt, if you like. Drink 4 to 6 oz. five to seven times throughout the day. This will soothe your intestinal tract and helps you absorb nutrients.

Rice water, made from brown rice, is much better than using white rice, unless you are allergic to it. It will help you firm up loose stools and replace your body's B vitamins. These vitamins are carried out of your body in your watery stools.

Make brown rice water by combining half-cup of rice to 3 cups of boiling water. Simmer for 45 minutes. Strain out the rice, to eat later, and drink the remaining rice water. Drink this water 3 to 4 times a day.

Yogurt, Bananas & Applesauce

Consume yogurt with bananas or cooked applesauce to get some fiber. This is soothing and is high in pectin, which calms the intestinal tract and replaces nutrients that diarrhea rinses out - magnesium and potassium.

Acute Diarrhea

When you have Acute Diarrhea, you need to stop eating regular food, and this is essential. This will rest your intestinal tract. When you have diarrhea and you eat food, this food will not be properly digested and will turn into toxic acid and cause you more stomach problems.

Charcoal Tablets

Take 4 charcoal tablets every hour for 3 to 4 hours, and then reduce to three times a day for two more days, or until the diarrhea stops. The charcoal will make your stools black. Check your health-food store for these tablets.

When using charcoal tablets, don't take them with food or vitamins. When you don't have or can't get charcoal tablets, eat a well burnt piece of toast.

Water Therapy

To avoid dehydration with diarrhea, drink water throughout the day.

Here is a way to stop diarrhea, when it is an emergency to do so. This should only be done by a person, who was normally healthy before the diarrhea. It should not be done by sickly children, weak elderly, pregnant women, or people with heart problems.

Create a sitz bath of 6 to 8 inches of cold water and ½ cup of apple cider vinegar. Sit in the bath for a few seconds and increase the time gradually to 10 minutes. The temperature should be 40F to 50 F.

To avoid drafts, cover your back and chest with dry towels. Have someone to massage your upper body through towels.

When you have completed the bath, get a massage over your entire body with a rough towel.

Children Chronic Diarrhea Attack

When your child has diarrhea, try to determine the cause and eliminate the cause.

You can use the water therapy mentioned above for healthy children, except use it as follows. This water therapy will strengthen your child's digestive and immune system.
In the bathroom without a draft, sit your child in cold water up to their waist, for a few seconds at a time. Then, dry them and do this every day for only a few seconds, and do this for a week, if necessary.

3: Foods That Cure the Good Diarrhea

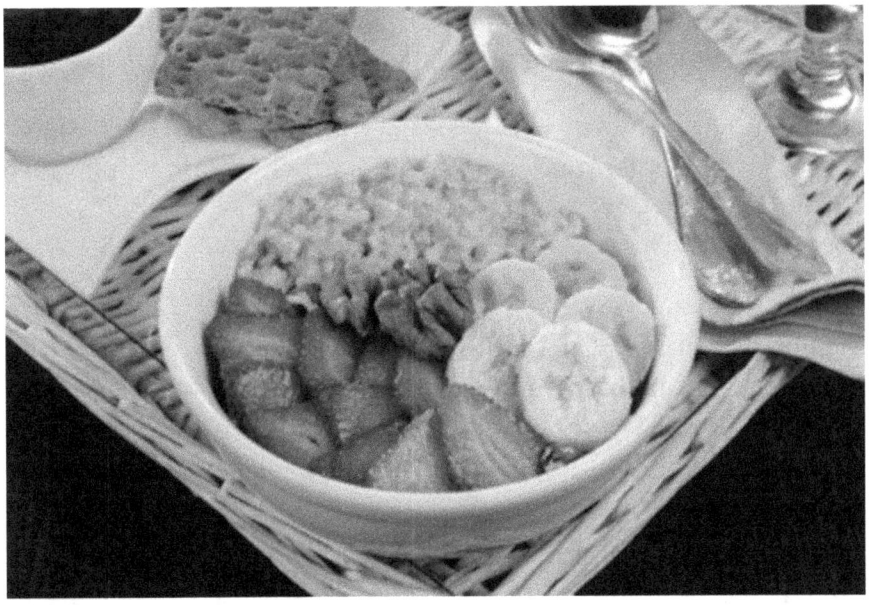

These are the foods that you can eat when you have diarrhea. These foods will help you recover quicker from this condition. Use these foods throughout the day. You can use other similar foods, but, these are the basics.

Apple and Pectin

Apples are good for digestion. It can relieve both diarrhea and constipation. Apples have pectin a soluble fiber.

For diarrhea, eat the outer skin of the apple. If you have dried apple peels, simmering them in warm water will help regulate your digestion. For maximum benefit, eat 1 to 2 medium-sized apples every day.

Apples are high in potassium, and this mineral is lost in large amount when you have diarrhea.

Pectin

Pectin is the soluble fiber found in fruits and vegetables. It is a thickening agent that is used to make jams and jellies. It is an excellent remedy for diarrhea.

A homemade way to get extra pectin is to make applesauce. Cook some apples and mash them up. Eat this applesauce throughout the day.

Bananas

Bananas will help you eliminate diarrhea. In your colon, bananas will absorb water, so that your stool will not be so watery. Bananas are also high in potassium, which is used to replenish the potassium lost during your diarrhea.

Bananas should not be used with some people with diarrhea.

Blueberry

Blueberries are a common Swedish folk remedy for diarrhea, and they also fight infections and kill bacteria and viruses. They are known for clearing up most cases of diarrhea. Here's what to do.

Eat fresh or frozen berries three times daily or half a cup of blueberry juice in the morning and at night. If you have blueberry leaves, you can make a tea of the leaves.

Use one tablespoon of leaves and simmer in half a cup of hot water. Strain the tea and drink.

If you can get **bilberry** extract at your health-food store, then add sixteen drops of the extract to a cup of chamomile or peppermint tea.

Coconut Macaroons

Coconut Macaroons may be helpful for your diarrhea. These cookies are high in fiber, fat and contain modified starch, egg white, soy lecithin, sweeteners, and coconut.

Milk and Cinnamon

Here is a diarrhea remedy that is made by adding two pinches of cinnamon and one pinch of cloves into a cup of warm milk. Make sure you are not lactose intolerant, if you use this remedy. You can also use Rice Dream milk or almond milk as a substitute for milk.

Oats and Cream of Wheat

Here is a remedy that is easy, and you should have the ingredients in your cupboard. Mix up some oats or cream of wheat, milk with a pinch of cinnamon, and add some blueberries, raspberries, or bananas. This will decrease your diarrhea condition within three hours and reduce the time you have diarrhea by 50%. You can also use the milks mentioned in the previous chapter, rice dream milk, or almond milk.

Egg Yolk

Using egg yolk is a time-tested remedy for children. You can prepare soft or hard-boiled eggs for children with diarrhea.

Carrots

Carrot juice and carrot soup are great cures for diarrhea. Here's what to do.

Drink two glasses of carrot juice. Preparing your own carrot juice is a good idea, since it will have more fiber than store bought.

You can make a carrot soup and sip about a pint during the day. Just cut up a good amount of carrots and boil them under low heat for about an hour. Then drink the water.

Raspberry

To use raspberry for diarrhea, take one ounce of raspberry leaves and steeped in 20 ounces of hot water for fifteen minutes, strained, and drink two cups per day. Drink the tea cold.

If you have fresh or frozen berries, eat them throughout the day or first thing in the morning and evening.

Vegetable Broth

Create a vegetable broth with ½ cup of brown rice. Cut up whole unpeeled potatoes and vegetables, such as carrots, onions, and celery. Put them in a pot of water and cook for two to three hours, then strain. Sip this healing broth, throughout the day.

Apricots

Eat apricots to give you fiber and minerals to replace these nutrients that are expelled during your diarrhea.

Banana Smoothie

Blend banana, un-sweeten yogurt, one teaspoon of organic applesauce, and a pinch of cinnamon with adequate water to make a pleasant consistency.

As your diarrhea condition improves, start eating some carbohydrates.

End of Diarrhea

When your diarrhea is gone, eat fresh papaya, fresh pineapple and their fresh juices to replace digestive enzymes that have been flushed out of your body by your diarrhea. Also, drink some lemon juice, without sugar to put back some minerals into your body.

Solid Food

Here is a list of solid foods that you should be eating as soon as you see your diarrhea is decreasing.

Yogurt without sugar, carrots, celery, spinach, beetroot, cranberries, blueberries, banana, ginger, carrot juice, mashed potatoes

4: Juices That Are Good for diarrhea

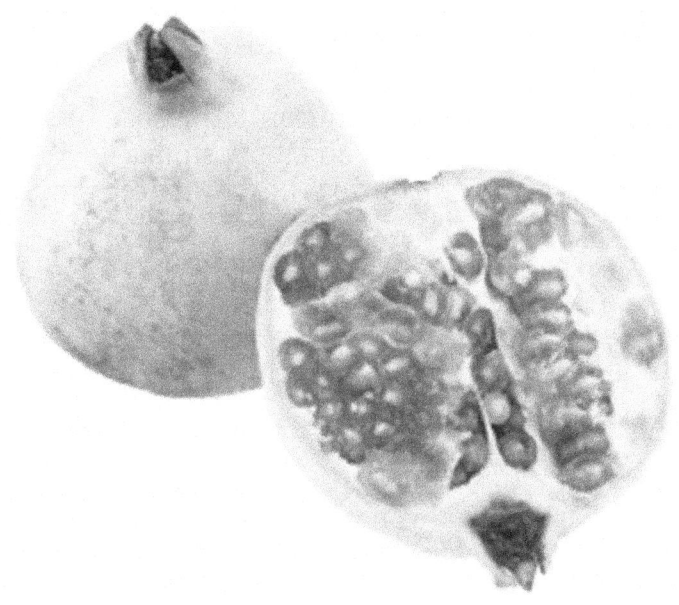

Drinking juices for diarrhea

When you have diarrhea, don't drink any raw juices until your diarrhea has reduced in intensity. Then, you can drink juices, especially papaya juice, lemon juice, fresh pineapple juice.

Use these juices to fight the dehydration that results from diarrhea and for the replacement of minerals and nutrients that you have lost.

Honey Drink

Mix half a teaspoon of honey with a pinch of salt into an 8-ounce glass of fresh orange, apple, or other fruit juice. Now, make another drink with ¼ teaspoon baking soda into a separate 8-ounce glass of water. You can alternate drinking these beverages, until they're finished.

Quince Juice

The juice of quince has been found to stop acute diarrhea. This juice is an astringent and is sour. You can try to add a few drop of honey, to make it more tolerable. However, if you use it without the honey, this is the way to use it.

Use the green fruit or un-ripen fruit to make your juice. You should only take 1/2 a cup on an empty stomach. You can use up to a maximum of 1 cup during the day, if necessary.

Pomegranate

You can use the whole fruit and rind for diarrhea. If you can find fresh juice, drink three glasses during the day.

Rhubarb Juice Powder

If you have diarrhea that is not caused by a bacterial infection, you can use one tablespoon of rhubarb powder mixed in one glass of water.

5: Remedies That Cure Diarrhea

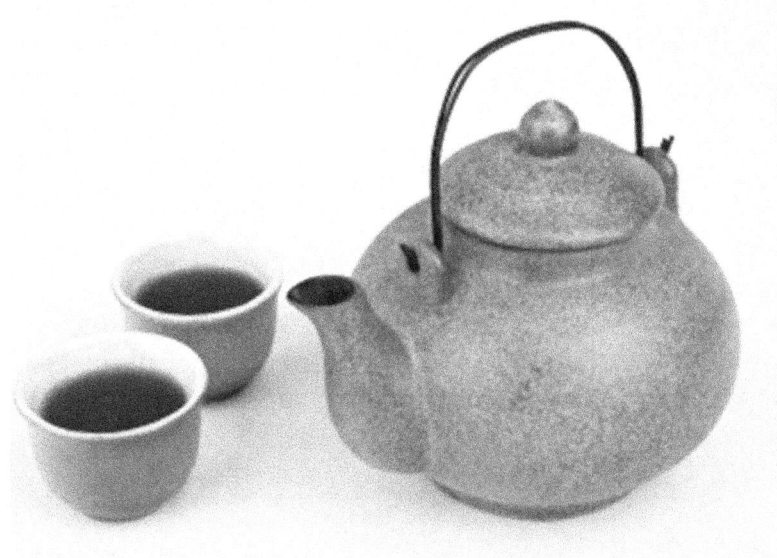

Here are some natural remedies that you need to use to get rid of your diarrhea.

Aloe Vera Drink

Drink One cup of liquid aloe vera one to two times a day in between meals. Liquid aloe vera can be purchased at a health-food store.

Slippery Elm

Slippery elm can stop mild diarrhea quickly. Here's what to do.

Heat some water and place 1 big teaspoon of powdered slippery elm into the water. You can also put it into a glass of warm juice. Drink this mixture and continue to drink two to three more glasses every 1/2 hour. This should stop your diarrhea.

Or you can use 1 ounce powdered slippery elm in 1 quart boiling water, which is simmered down to a pint. Then, take one teaspoon every ½ hour, to soothe the membranes of the intestinal tract. Use honey to make this tea taste better.

Oregon Graperoot

Oregon graperoot, goldenseal, and barberry herb can fight and kill a broad range of microbes, such as shigella, salmonella, E. coli, and V. cholera, and the parasite giardia. Because of this, it is effective for diarrhea.

Make a tea out of Oregon graperoot or combine all three herbs and make a tea from them. Drink 2-3 cups during the day.

Basil

Use a decoction of basil with honey and nutmeg for diarrhea.

Bilberry

Typical dosage: 2 or 3 capsules or tablets, standardized to 25 percent anthocyanosides, per day.

Black Tea

Drink black tea with a slight amount of honey.
Do this for around two hours to get control of your diarrhea. Now, eat a couple spoonful of un-sweeten yogurt, every few hours and also continue to drink the black tea.

Carob Powder

You can use roasted carob powder to get relief from diarrhea. This powder is high in fiber and contains polyphenols, which help reduce diarrhea.

Cascarilla bark

Make an infusion of this herb and take a tablespoon at a time. For the infusion, put one ounce of the herb into one pint of boiling water, steep for 20 minutes and then strain.

Catnip

Catnip is a mild sedative, good for cramps, and upset stomach. It has been used in Europe for diarrhea. Drink this tea to control your diarrhea.

Catnip has a mild sedative effect and is useful for cramps and upset stomach. In Europe, this herb is a popular diarrhea remedy.

For catnip capsules: Take 1 to 3 daily
For catnip extract: In 1/2 cup warmed water, add ½ to 1 teaspoon of catnip and drink it.

Ginger Oil

Use ginger oil or ginger root tea. For the oil, add one drop into a glass of warm water and drink. You can also make a tea of ginger root and drink. Drink this tea throughout the day.

Goldenseal

Goldenseal fights infections prevents and relieves diarrhea. It is known for treating microbial infections. You can buy them in capsule, but make sure you don't use them in excess, since they may create diarrhea; the very thing you are trying to eliminate.

Grapefruit Seed oil

Grapefruit seed oil is considered an alternative to pharmaceutical antibiotics. You can get it in pill form and eliminate candida, which can create diarrhea.

Herbal Teas

Here are some other herbal teas to drink, when you have diarrhea – chamomile, yarrow, and nettle.

Make a strong tea of slippery elm, peppermint, red raspberry, and ½ teaspoon cinnamon. Sip the tea throughout the day. If you don't have all these teas, use the ones you have.

Lungwort

As its name suggests, this herb is good for coughs, hoarseness, and mild lung problems. It can also be used for diarrhea, which makes it the herb of choice for stomach virus accompanied by a cough. Here's how to use it. Mix 1 tablespoon dry herb into 1 cup hot water. Drink 1 cup daily.

Peppermint oil

Peppermint oil is used to aid digestion, abdominal pain, bloating, frequent bowel movements, and diarrhea.

You can buy enteric capsule and take them as directed.

6: Supplements Good for Diarrhea

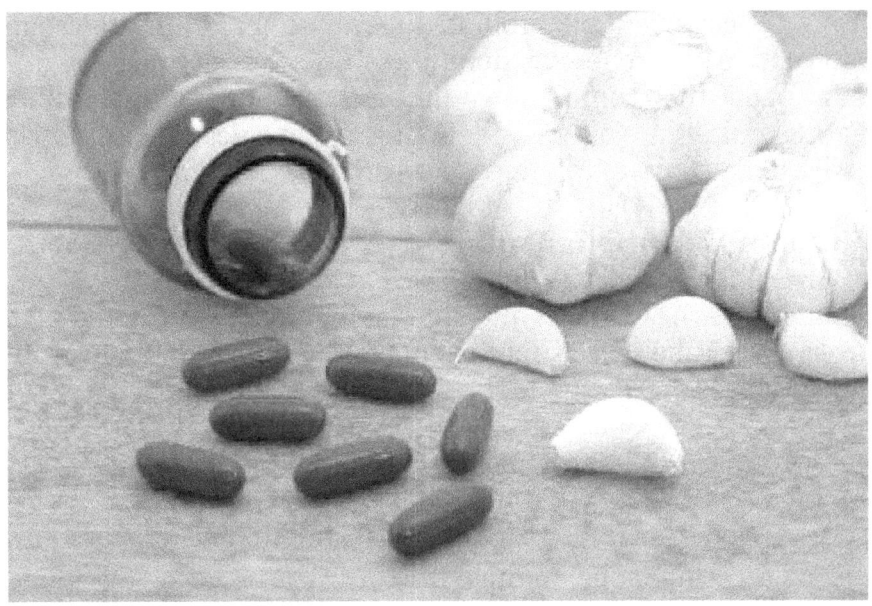

Nutrient deficiencies

When you are low in certain nutrients, which protect the intestinal lining and gastrointestinal tract, this may cause diarrhea. You don't want to be short on zinc, vitamin A, niacin, folic acid, and B1,B3, and glutamine.

Probiotics

You need to take probiotics during and after your bout with diarrhea. This will help to rebalance your intestinal good bacteria-Lactobacillus acidophilus, Bifidobacteria bifidum, and Lactobacillus bulgaricus, Take a dose of from one billion to ten billion of these good bacteria daily.

Take a capsules, liquid, or powdered of Lactobacillus

acidophilus, and Lactobacillus bulgaricus. These good bacteria combat diarrhea-inducing bacteria, E. coli, salmonella, streptococci, and shigella.

Take 4 capsules of probiotics four times a day. As an alternative, eat generous amounts of un-sweeten milk, goat, or soy yogurt that contains live probiotics. You should continue eating cultured yogurt and taking 2 capsules of probiotics twice a day, for two to three weeks after having diarrhea.

Vitamins & Supplements

Here is a list of vitamins and supplements that you should take every day. Take these supplements for at least 4 weeks or until you get your diarrhea under control.

- Vitamin C – 200 mg. every hour for about 8 hours
- Aged Garlic – Use capsules and double the amount recommended on the bottle.
- Pepsin tablets or comfrey-pepsin tablets
- Pulverized charcoal – 1 tsp. or 3 tablets every 2 hours
- Take vitamin A, 10,000 IU
- Take Zinc picolinate, 30 mg
- Take B50 or B100 supplement to get all the B vitamins

When you have vomiting or stomach issues, it's best not to use supplements. Wait until these issues are corrected.

If you have not been eating a good diet, you should be taking a multivitamin and multimineral supplement.

After Diarrhea Supplements

After you have eliminated your diarrhea, you should take the following supplements to rebuild your intestinal lining and replacing your digestive enzymes and good bacteria. This will help you strengthen your immune system, so that you do not have a recurrence of diarrhea, in your near future.

Take the following for one month.

- Deglycyrrhizinated licorice (DGL). Take two 380 mg tablets by chewing them 20 minutes before meals, three or four times a day. This coats, soothes, and helps rejuvenate intestinal lining.

- Glutamine. 500-mg two times a day

- N-acetyl-D-glucosamine. 500 mg two to four times a day.

- Take potassium, 100 mg and a multi-mineral supplement

- Take garlic capsules for their antibiotic impact during or after meals.

Medical Supplements and pills

Here are some of the medicines that are prescribed when you have diarrhea.

- Bismuth subsalicylate is a form of Pepto-Bismol, which cuts down the secretion of the intestines and turns your stools black.

- Loperamide (Immodium) or diphenoxylate (Lomotil), slows down your intestine movement and their secretions. However, they may worsen your condition, by slowing down the evacuation responsible organisms.

- Kaopectate, which is a Nonabsorbable earth mixtures of kaolin and pectin, makes your stools bulky.

7: A Plan For Eliminating Diarrhea

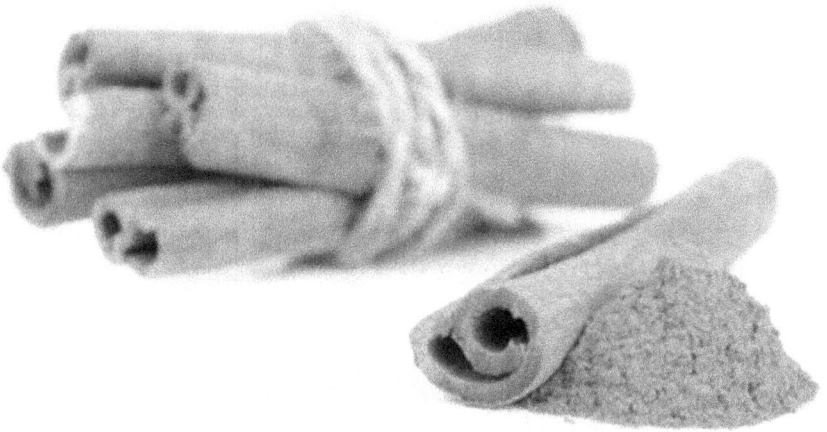

Diarrhea can turn into a serious condition, which can lead to other diseases, because of nutritional deficiency. Here is a plan for you to start out with, so that you can reduce and eliminate your diarrhea.

Regardless of the cause of your diarrhea, you can start out by assuming that it was caused by some type of bacteria or viral food contamination. When you do this, you will be using those remedies that target any food contamination from pathogens or poisons.

If you have acute diarrhea and need to get relief quickly, then consider using a sitz bath as outline in chapter 2.

Step one – do not eat the food you normally eat or drink any fruit or vegetable juices at this point.

Step two - make rice water as outlined in chapter 2. The water in this rice drink will keep you hydrated. Make sure you use the various tea and drinks provided here, to keep hydrated. Use this rice water in place of other recipes that call for milk. You can also use Rice Dream milk.

Step three – go to chapter 3 and eat those foods listed there for breakfast lunch and dinner.

Step four – go to chapter 4 and use Quince Juice, if you can find it at your health-food store or Internet.

Step five – Go to chapter 5 and pick out the best teas to make between meals. Start with Slippery elm tea. Make a Oregon Graperoot tea and try some roasted carob.

Step six – go to chapter 6 and see if you have some of the vitamins and mineral mentioned there. For sure, take the B50 vitamins, zinc, and potassium.

Step seven – during your bout with diarrhea make sure you are taking good bacteria in the form of pills or un-sweeten yogurt.

As your diarrhea starts to lessen, you can follow this recommendation, "When your diarrhea is less or gone, eat fresh papaya, fresh pineapple and their fresh juices to replace digestive enzymes that have been flushed out of your body, by your diarrhea. Also, drink some lemon juice, without sugar to put back some minerals into your body."

Step eight – when you feel your diarrhea is gone, take the follow supplements and nutrients for a month.

"Deglycyrrhizinated licorice (DGL). Take two 380 mg tablets by chewing them 20 minutes before meals three or four times a day. This coats, soothes, and helps rejuvenate intestinal lining."

"Take 4 - capsules of probiotics four times a day. As an alternative, eat generous amounts of un-sweeten milk, goat, soy yogurt, or plain yogurt that contains live probiotics."

Step nine - Take garlic capsules for their antibiotic impact during or after meals.

Step ten - eat the solid foods listed in chapter 3:

Yogurt without sugar, carrots, celery, spinach, beetroot, cranberries, blueberries, banana, ginger, carrot juice, mashed potatoes

There you have it. You have a lot of different remedies and supplements to use and you don't have to use all of them. Just pick a few to work with, as I have outlined above.

Use the remedies and foods that are available to you and that you feel comfortable using. Some of the drinks and teas may not taste as good as you like, but consider them a remedy that can cure your condition.

Most of these remedies have been found effective for different levels of diarrhea. They do not work for all people that is why I have been giving you many remedies, so that if one or two remedies don't work for you, you have others you can choose from.

Use as many of the supplements listed here, since they will help you replenished the nutrients you lost during your diarrhea condition.

Chapter 6: About The Author And Other Resources

Get one of my best kindle books *free* below:

http://www.natural-remedies-thatwork.com

Rudy Silva is a natural nutritional consultant educated in the United States in Nutrition and Physics. He is a graduate from San Jose State University in California. He is author of 45 other books on natural remedies. He has authored a newsletter in natural remedies for over 10 years.

Resource page

Here are some of the other kindle e-books about natural remedies that have been written by this author. You can see the entire list at:

http://tinyurl.com/b2f7wd3

Acne Remedies

- Best natural acne treatments: Acne facial
- Effective Acne Treatments That Work

Constipation Remedies

- The Best Constipation Remedies
- Best Constipated Women Natural Cures
- How To Relieve Constipation With Fruits

Essential Fatty Acids

- Taking The Mystery Out Of Essential Fatty acids

- Amazing Fish Oil Benefits Revealed
- Omega 3 and 6 Mystery Exposed

Nutrition Remedies

- Updated Version - Secret Diet And Nutrition
- Secret Healthy Fruit Practices Revealed
- Fast Healing Juice Nutrition Therapy: Nutrition Tips 3
- Fantastic Alkaline Fruit Benefits Revealed
- Calcium (Discover How To Use Calcium To Avoid Devastating Diseases)
- Magnesium Nutrition Revealed
- Best Nutrition Health Practices
- Potassium Health Secrets Revealed
- Phosphorus, The Best Brain Food
- A Sodium Diet (What You Must Know About Sodium)
- Vegetables and Vegetable Juice Cures
- Alkaline Body: How to Change an Acid Body into an Alkaline body

Stomach Remedies

- Acid Reflux: Fast and Easy Cures For Acid Reflux
- Asthma Treatment Cures With Remedies
- How To Do Natural Colon Cleansing
- Gastrointestinal Digestion Secrets Revealed

Misc Remedies

- Natural Hair Loss Treatment: Women And Men
- Effective Natural Hemorrhoids Treatment
- Iron Deficiency Anemia
- Secrets To Understanding Behavior
- Fast Acting Ear Infection Remedies
- Best Behavior Secrets Revealed That Can Change Your Personality

- What Is A Hiatus Hernia
- Best Varicose Vein Treatments?
- Make Shampoos At Home Using Natural Ingredients:Discover recipes for quality natural hair shampoos
- How To Fix Your Thyroid Problems: Discover Hidden Ideas That Fix Your Thyroid

Minerals

- Calcium and Magnesium Magic Body Benefits Revealed
- The Magic of Sodium, Calcium and Magnesium
- Create an Alkaline Body with Potassium and Sodium: Eliminate a Potassium Deficiency
- Calcium and Phosphorus Foods: Deficiency or Excesses in These Minerals Cause Bone and Brain Power Loss
- Chlorine The Body Detoxifier (With water, chlorine will clean your body of toxins and pathogens)

Men's Health

- Best Impotence Health Diet

Weight loss

- Ten (10) Day Quick Success Weight Loss Program: A new approach to losing weight by changing your eating habits for life
- Discover Secret Anti-Aging Juice & Tonic Recipes: Unique Juices And Tonics That Create Beauty And Youth

To see all the kindle books written by this author, go to this the Authors Profile Page or this URL: http://tinyurl.com/b2f7wd3

If you need support or want to promote any of his e-books,

please contact him at rss41@yahoo.com and expect a reply within 24 hours. He looks forward to hearing from you and is happy to help you understand his material on natural and nutritional health.

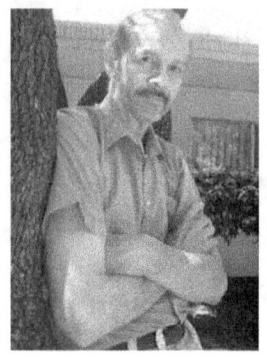

Give A Review

And, don't for get to give a review for this e-book at Amazon so that others can gain the benefits of what is in this e-book. To you, for losing weight, creating better health and more happiness in your life,

Rudy S Silva